10-05
J 616.853

Understanding Diseases and Disorders

Epilepsy

Hayley Mitchell Haugen

12139887

KIDHAVEN PRESS
An imprint of Thomson Gale, a part of The Thomson Corporation

Fowlerville District Library

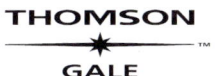

Detroit • New York • San Francisco • San Diego • New Haven, Conn. • Waterville, Maine • London • Munich

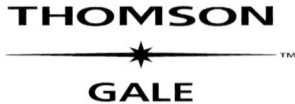

© 2005 Thomson Gale, a part of The Thomson Corporation.

Thomson and Star Logo are trademarks and Gale and KidHaven Press are registered trademarks used herein under license.

For more information, contact
KidHaven Press
27500 Drake Rd.
Farmington Hills, MI 48331-3535
Or you can visit our Internet site at http://www.gale.com

ALL RIGHTS RESERVED.
No part of this work covered by the copyright hereon may be reproduced or used in any form or by any means—graphic, electronic, or mechanical, including photocopying, recording, taping, Web distribution or information storage retrieval systems—without the written permission of the publisher.

Every effort has been made to trace the owners of copyrighted material.

Picture Credits: Cover photo: © Owen Franken/CORBIS; © Jeff Albertson/CORBIS, 11; AP/Wide World Photos, 38; Jeff Christensen/Reuters/Landov, 27; CNRI/Photo Researchers, Inc., 14; © Alan Goldsmith/CORBIS, 18; © Hulton-Deutsch Collection/CORBIS, 9; Issei Kato/Reuters/Landov, 16; Chris Jouan, 17, 37; Erich Lessing/Art Resource, NY, 21; © Lawrence Manning/CORBIS, 28; PhotoDisc, 23; Photos.com, 5, 8, 24, 33 (both); © Antonia Reeve/Photo Researchers, Inc., 31; © Roger Ressmeyer/CORBIS, 34

LIBRARY OF CONGRESS CATALOGING-IN-PUBLICATION DATA

Haugen, Hayley Mitchell.
 Epilepsy / by Hayley Mitchell Haugen.
  v. cm. — (Understanding diseases and disorders)
 Includes bibliographical references and index.
 Contents: What is epilepsy?—What causes epilepsy?—Living with epilepsy—Treating epilepsy.
  ISBN 0-7377-2168-5 (hbk. : alk. paper)
  I. Title. II. Series. (San Diego, Calif.)

Printed in the United States of America

Contents

Chapter 1
What Is Epilepsy? 4

Chapter 2
What Causes Epilepsy? 13

Chapter 3
Living with Epilepsy 20

Chapter 4
Treating Epilepsy 30

Notes 40

Glossary 42

For Further Exploration 44

Index 47

Chapter One

What Is Epilepsy?

The cerebral cortex is the part of the brain that controls lots of daily functions. Like a computer, the cerebral cortex sends electrical messages along its network of nerve cells, known as **neurons**. These messages process what people think, how they feel, and what they do each day. One disorder that affects how the cerebral cortex functions is **epilepsy**.

For most people, the electrical messages sent along the neurons are organized and efficient. For epileptics (people who have epilepsy), however, the electrical charges are not always under control. Sometimes, the neurons fire off faster than normal, in little bursts of electricity. Like scrambled signals sent through crossed telephone wires, these bursts of electricity cause the brain to send mixed-up messages to the body. When this happens, a person has an epileptic **seizure**.

During a seizure, an epileptic may have a range of symptoms. Some are minor, such as lip smacking, staring into space, or arm and leg jerking. Epileptic seizures can also make a person's vision blurry or cause a brief loss of hearing. In the worst epileptic seizures, a person may fall to the ground in **convulsions** and even pass out.

Whatever the effect of an epileptic seizure may be, however, it only lasts for a few seconds, or a few minutes at most. Once a seizure has passed, the neurons return to normal and the person with epilepsy can often return to his or her usual activities after a short rest.

Staring into space is one of the more mild symptoms of an epileptic seizure.

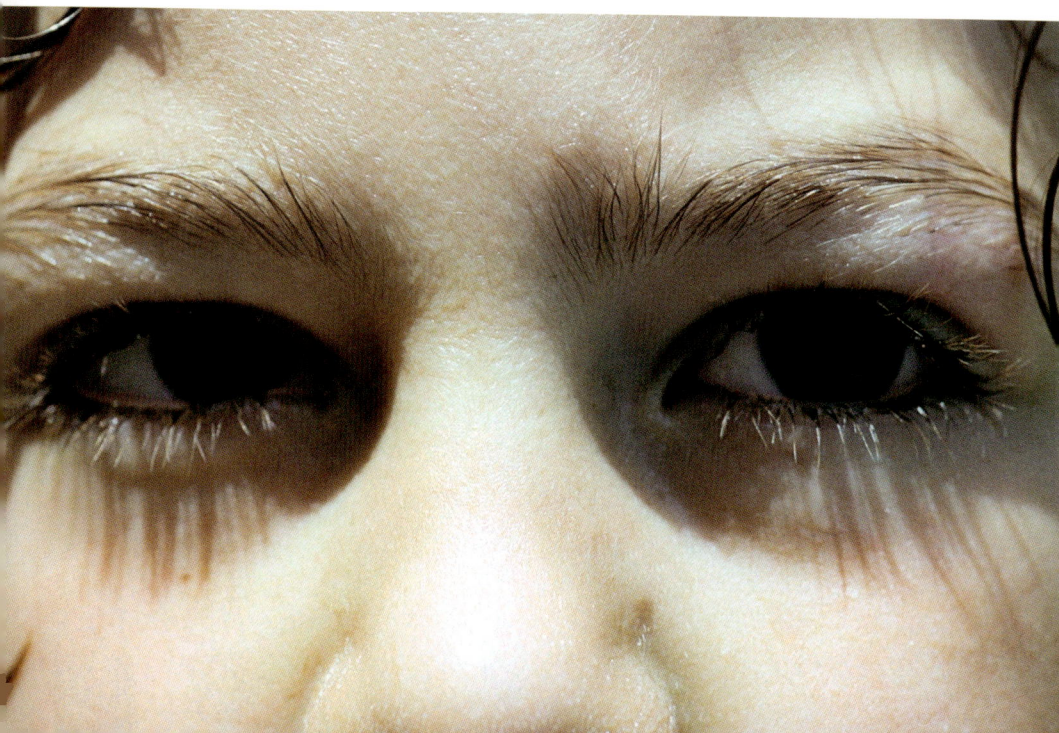

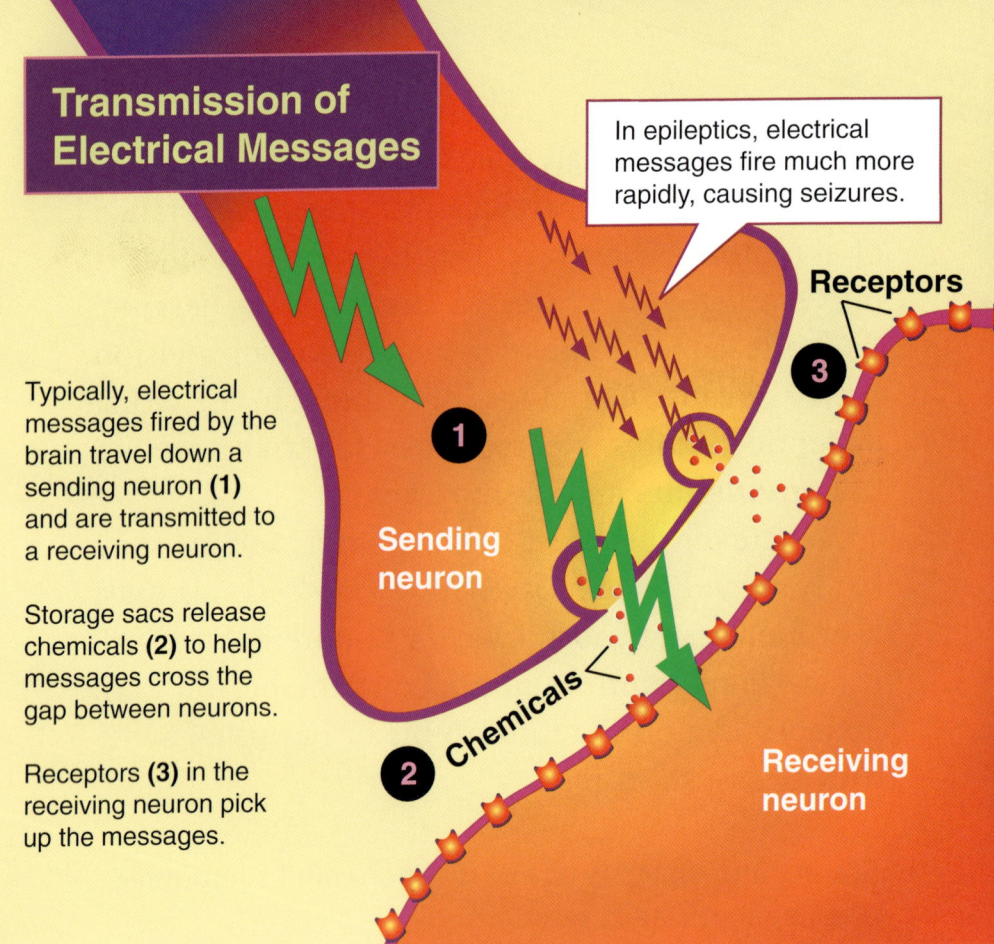

Ben is a boy in England who has epilepsy. The first time he had a seizure he was eight years old and playing soccer in his friend's front yard. Ben's vision got blurry, and he says his friend Jonathan sounded as if he were miles away. The next thing Ben knew, he was waking up in Jonathan's kitchen. "I asked him to tell me what happened to me after I started to feel weird," Ben remembers. "He said I just stopped running and then went all kind of stiff and fell over. Then my arms and legs jerked a bit and then I was just unconscious."[1]

In addition to affecting the body, as in Ben's case, epilepsy can also influence a person's emotions. During an attack, epileptics might suddenly feel sad at happy occasions, for example, or they might become loud and boisterous at solemn ones.

Who Has Epilepsy?

Epilepsy is not a rare disorder. The Epilepsy Foundation reports that 2.3 million Americans have epilepsy. About 300,000 of these people are children ages fourteen or younger. About 181,000 people are diagnosed with epilepsy each year.

Epilepsy can affect both young and old, male and female, and people of every race. Many disorders are inherited conditions, passed down from mothers and fathers to their children. This is true with epilepsy. Parents with epilepsy are more likely to have children with the disorder than parents who do not have it.

Medical research has also discovered that males are a little more likely to have epilepsy than females, but doctors have not learned why. What is known is that although epilepsy can develop at any age, it is most common in people under age twenty or over age sixty-five. Those with the condition usually have their first seizures sometime during childhood. However, 68 to 93 percent of epileptic children grow out of the disorder within twenty years of their first seizures.

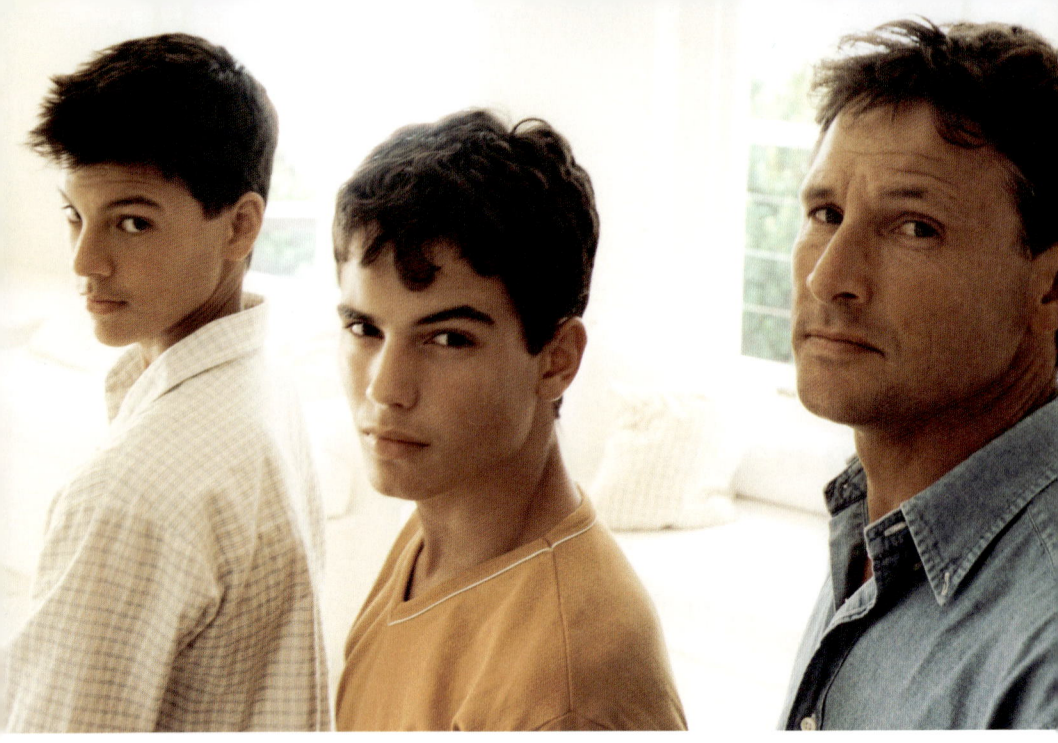

Although doctors are not certain why, males are more likely than females to have epilepsy.

What Does Epilepsy Do to People?

Epileptics can have over forty different types of seizures. These seizures fall into one of two categories: **partial seizures** or **generalized seizures**. Partial seizures occur in one area of the brain. Generalized seizures spread quickly throughout the brain, affecting more than one area at once.

Partial seizures are the most common. Since partial seizures only occur in one area of the brain at a time, only one area of the body is affected during the seizure. If a partial seizure occurs in the area that controls vision, for example, only the person's vision is affected by the seizure. Someone experiencing a visual seizure may have blurry vision or might see things that are not there. In the same way, partial seizures that occur in the area of the brain that controls hearing can cause people to hear voices, music, and other sounds that are not really there.

Unlike partial seizures, generalized seizures involve the whole brain. There are several types of generalized seizures. Two of the most common ones are **grand mal seizures** and **petit mal seizures**. People who experience grand mal seizures lose consciousness during their seizure. Their muscles contract, which can cause their body to thrash around while they are unconscious.

Grand mal seizures usually last from three to five minutes, but they take longer than that to

Doctors use a head device to test the electrical activity in an epileptic man's brain. This time-lapse photo shows the man has gone into a seizure during the test.

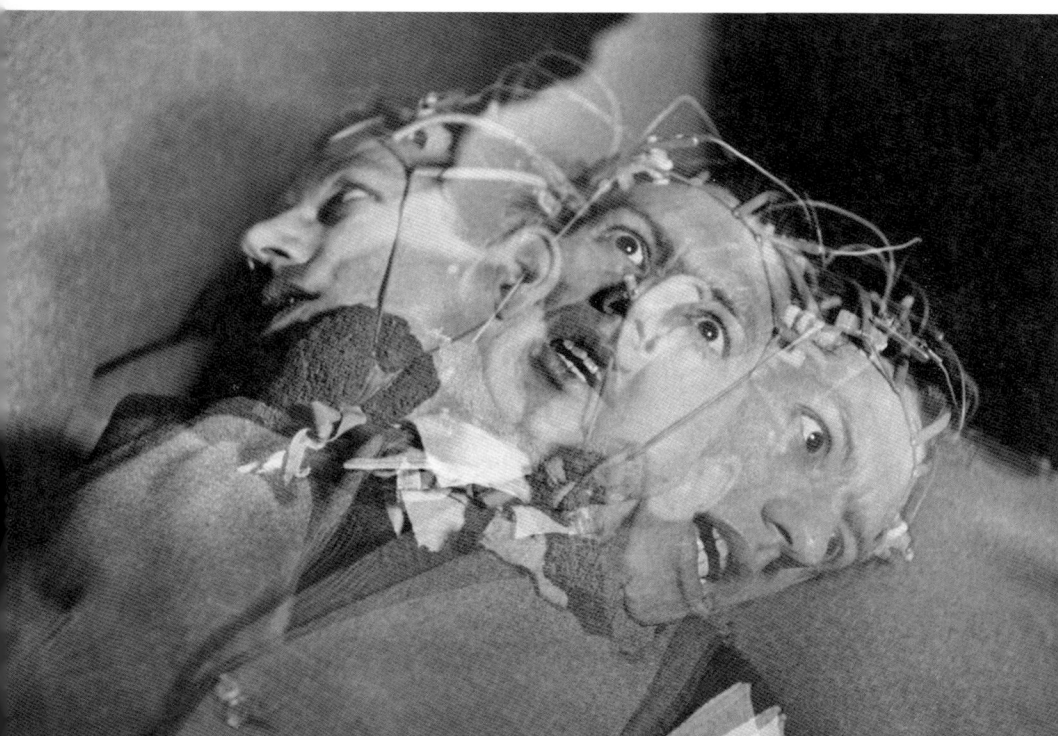

recover from. A person may remain unconscious for half an hour after an attack and may have no memory of the seizure upon awakening. Grand mal seizures can also leave behind headaches or muscle aches or weakness in the arms or legs.

Robert J. Michael, a teacher, describes his student Susan's grand mal seizure:

> Susan began to feel irritable and queasy. Her lips began to turn a purplish tone and she felt lightheaded. Her facial skin coloring lost its natural glow and became exceptionally pallid. Susan fell to the floor and lost consciousness. Her total body began to shake, twist, and writhe, and saliva began to drip slowly from the corner of her mouth. Her eyelids quivered, and it appeared that her eyes were rolled back. Several minutes later, she stopped convulsing and awoke, feeling quite tired and weary.[2]

Susan's experience is typical of grand mal seizures. For those who have petit mal seizures, the experience is less traumatic. The minds of people who have these seizures seem to tune out the world and become absent for brief moments throughout the day.

During petit mal seizures, which last about thirty seconds, a person may become very quiet, blink the eyes, stare into space, or simply pause

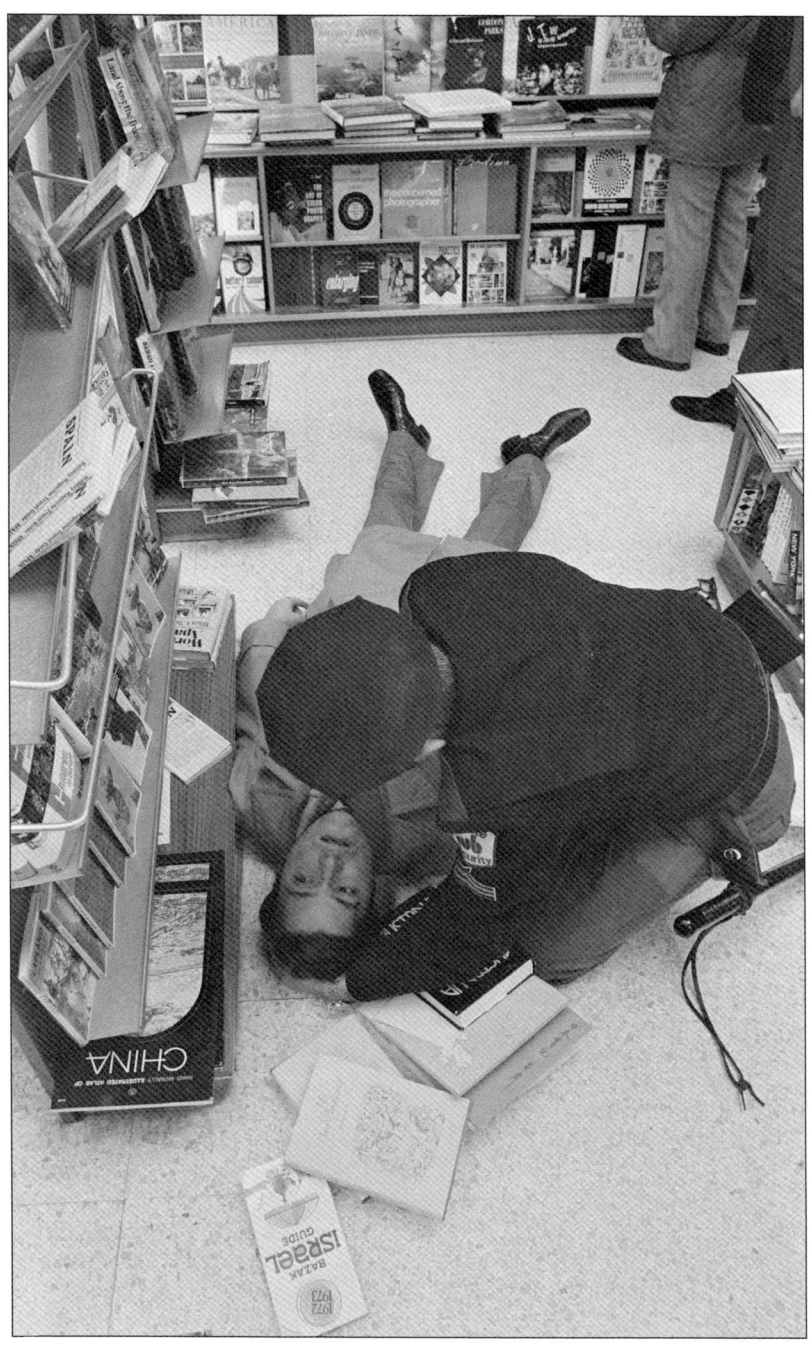

A police officer cradles the head of an epileptic having a seizure in a bookstore.

What Is Epilepsy? 11

during a conversation. Even though petit mal seizures cause people to lose consciousness for up to ten seconds, the signs of petit mal seizures are so small that people generally do not even know they are occurring. After the seizure they can simply return to whatever they were doing before the seizure occurred.

Although the effects of petit mal seizures are mild, without treatment a person who has these seizures can have as many as one hundred a day. These seizures can also lead to the more serious grand mal seizures. Fortunately for those who have epilepsy, doctors have found out a number of things that cause seizures. Epilepsy patients' experiences with seizures are unique, but each person can learn what activities cause him or her to have seizures.

Chapter Two

What Causes Epilepsy?

The cause of 50 to 70 percent of all cases of epilepsy is unknown. Doctors are able to find the causes of some cases, however. For example, 8 percent of epileptics inherit it from their parents. Sometimes epilepsy can occur as a result of trauma to a baby during childbirth. Lack of oxygen to the brain or an infection at birth, for instance, can cause the disorder.

Childhood diseases such as measles or mumps may cause seizures as well. Some poisons can also cause epilepsy. Lead in the paint in older homes is extremely poisonous. When lead paint chips are ingested by children, epilepsy, learning disorders, and in extreme cases, even death, can result. Mercury in thermometers and carbon monoxide in gasoline emissions are other poisons that can

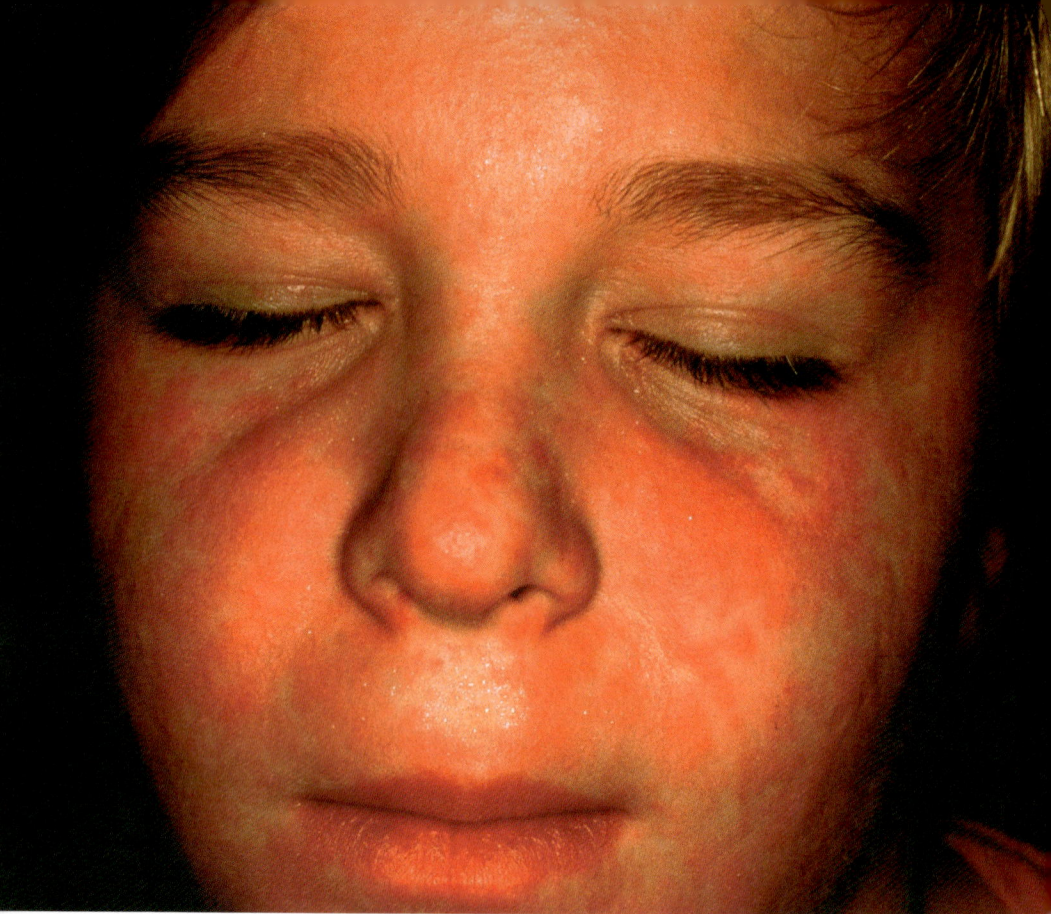

A child with measles breaks out in a rash. Measles can trigger seizures in some children.

cause epileptic seizures when swallowed or inhaled.

Injuries to the brain at any time of life can also cause epilepsy. People who injure their heads in severe car accidents or suffer gunshot wounds, for example, may develop seizures. Other medical conditions that affect the brain can also lead to epilepsy. **Strokes,** for example, prevent oxygen from getting to the brain. They are responsible for about 10 percent of epilepsy cases.

The elderly are more likely to have strokes than younger people. This explains why epilepsy increases after age sixty-five. Sometimes elderly people who experience stroke-related seizures never know it. Symptoms such as confusion and losing one's focus on things might be thought of as signs of aging, when in fact they may be epileptic seizures.

Certain Behaviors Can Trigger Seizures

Doctors cannot always detect the causes of a person's epilepsy, and for many people with the disorder, seizures also seem to have no cause. Others with the disorder, however, have been able to pinpoint things in their life that tend to cause seizures. These things are referred to as triggers.

About 5 percent of epileptics are sensitive to flickering lights. The condition is called photosensitivity. For these people, watching television and playing video games may trigger seizures. There are other triggers that affect a greater number of epileptics.

Stress and lack of sleep go hand in hand as two of the most common triggers of epileptic seizures. Catlina is an eighteen-year-old girl who developed epilepsy at age fifteen. In her case too many late nights and stressful, active days at school triggered her first seizures. She writes, "During that year I had unusual warning signs that something was

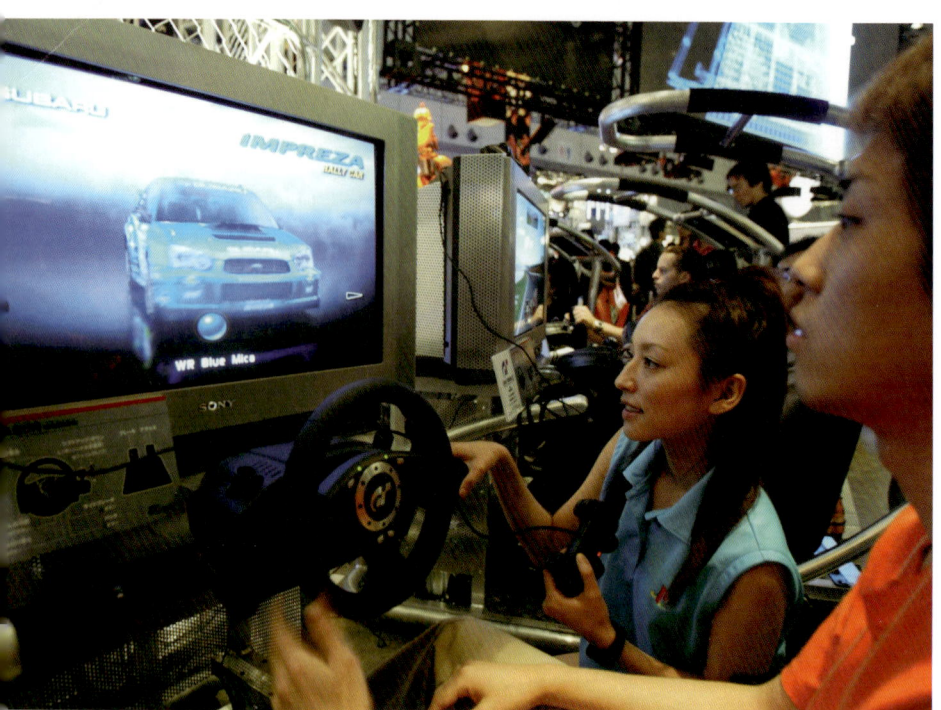

The flickering lights of video games are a seizure trigger for some epileptics.

wrong. In the mornings I'd get up after a late night to go to school that day, but my hands were jerking! I couldn't manage holding a cup of coffee right after I woke. I thought nothing of it."[3]

Catlina knew that she had not been eating regular meals, and she had been staying up later than normal to complete her school projects, but she did not know that her morning tremors were signs of epilepsy. Then one morning Catlina had a grand mal seizure. "I was in and out of consciousness from home to the hospital," she says. "I remember that the pants I was wearing were too big for me, so I kept on pulling them up in the ambulance! My mother and sister were in the ambulance too, crying hysterically. I thought I was going to die."[4]

In the hospital, Catlina learned she has epilepsy. The doctors started her on medication to control her seizures, and she has not suffered another grand mal seizure since. She says, however, that if she does not stay organized to help prevent stress at school, eat right, and try to get eight hours of sleep each night, her hands continue to shake in the mornings.

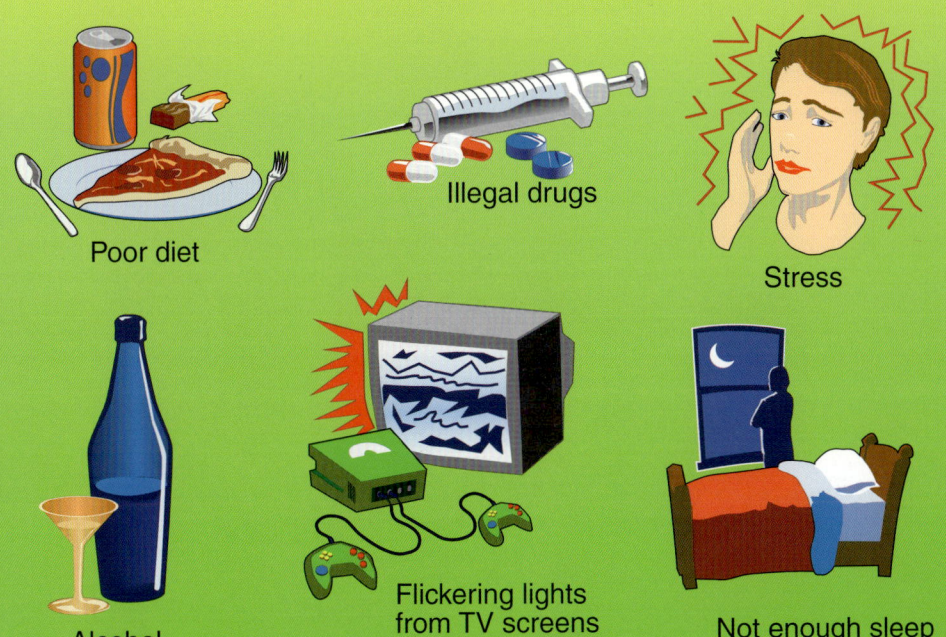

Triggers

In a person with epilepsy, these factors may trigger a seizure:

Poor diet

Illegal drugs

Stress

Alcohol

Flickering lights from TV screens and video games

Not enough sleep

Alcohol and Drugs Can Cause Seizures

Managing stress, eating regular meals, and getting lots of rest are all things that people like Catlina can do to help prevent epileptic seizures. There are also a number of things epileptics should not do, such as take drugs or drink too much alcohol. Alcohol and drugs both affect the nerve cells and neurons in the brain. Drinking beer, wine, or hard liquor can cause seizures even in people without epilepsy. Since epileptics are already affected by

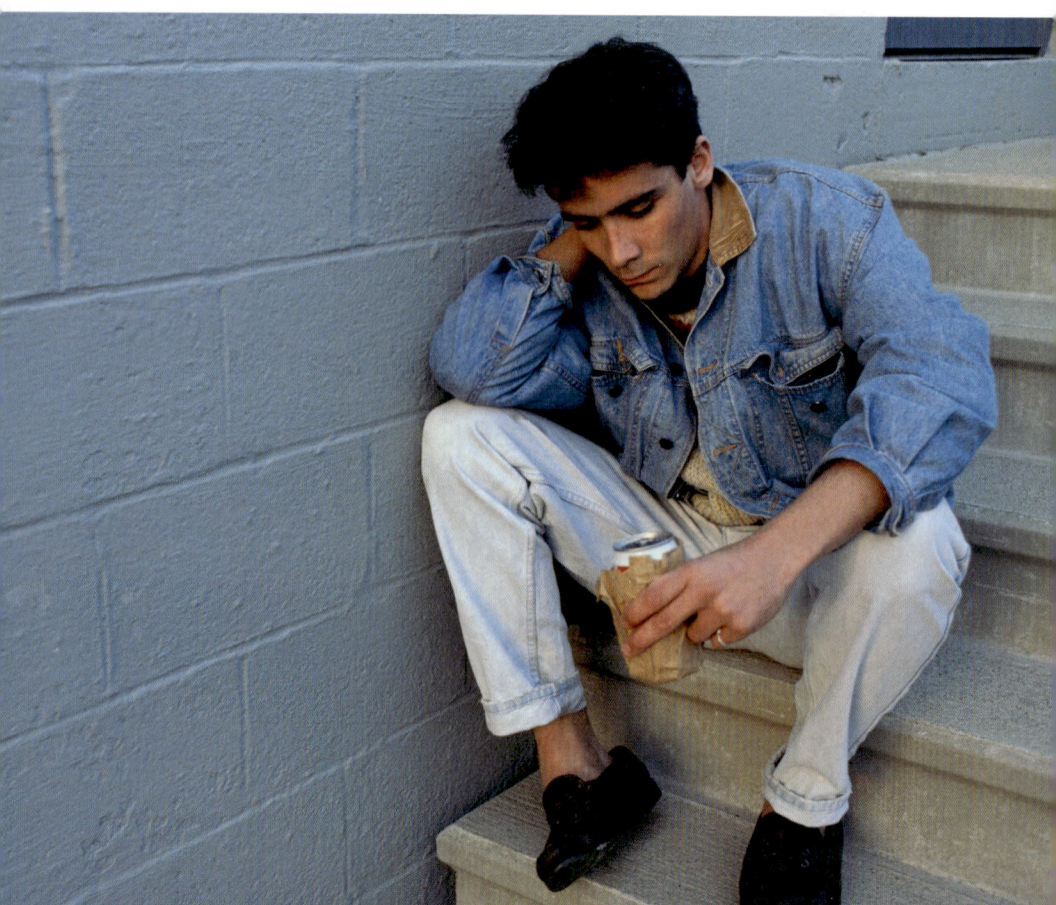

Because beer and liquor can trigger seizures, epileptics must limit how much alcohol they drink.

an abnormal functioning of nerve cells and neurons, alcohol and drugs can become triggers for seizures.

Because of this increased risk of seizures, it is important for epileptics not to take illegal drugs and not to drink more than one or two glasses of alcohol a day. Those on medication for their epilepsy should avoid alcohol entirely. Alcohol can make antiepileptic drugs less effective. Alcohol can also increase the negative side effects of epilepsy medication such as drowsiness or headaches.

Fortunately, alcohol consumption is a behavior people can control to prevent seizures. By learning what most often triggers their seizures, epileptics can modify their lifestyle and behaviors in all kinds of ways to help reduce epileptic episodes and live happily. Even people who have less control over their seizures because they do not know the causes of them are able to live happy, productive lives.

Chapter Three

Living with Epilepsy

Having epilepsy can affect the quality of a person's life in many ways. Some epileptics, for instance, have very few seizures each year. In others, the seizures are mild and easily controlled by limiting triggers. Epilepsy is also easier to manage for people who experience warning signals from their body that a seizure is coming on. A sudden change in vision, for example, may serve as a warning for a seizure. With this warning, people with epilepsy have time to make themselves comfortable in a safe place before their seizures strike.

Other epileptics, however, may have frequent or more severe seizures, and experience no warning signs before they hit. For these people, epilepsy is something they may fear daily. They may even have to wear helmets, or take other precautionary measures around their home.

Although the disorder is severe for some people, about 80 percent of epileptics can control the disorder either by taking medication or by avoiding triggers. There are few limits to what these epileptics can accomplish in their lives. In fact, a number of well-known epileptics have made extraordinary contributions to the world. Julius Caesar, Peter the Great, and Napoléon all had

French emperor Napoléon is one of history's most famous epileptics.

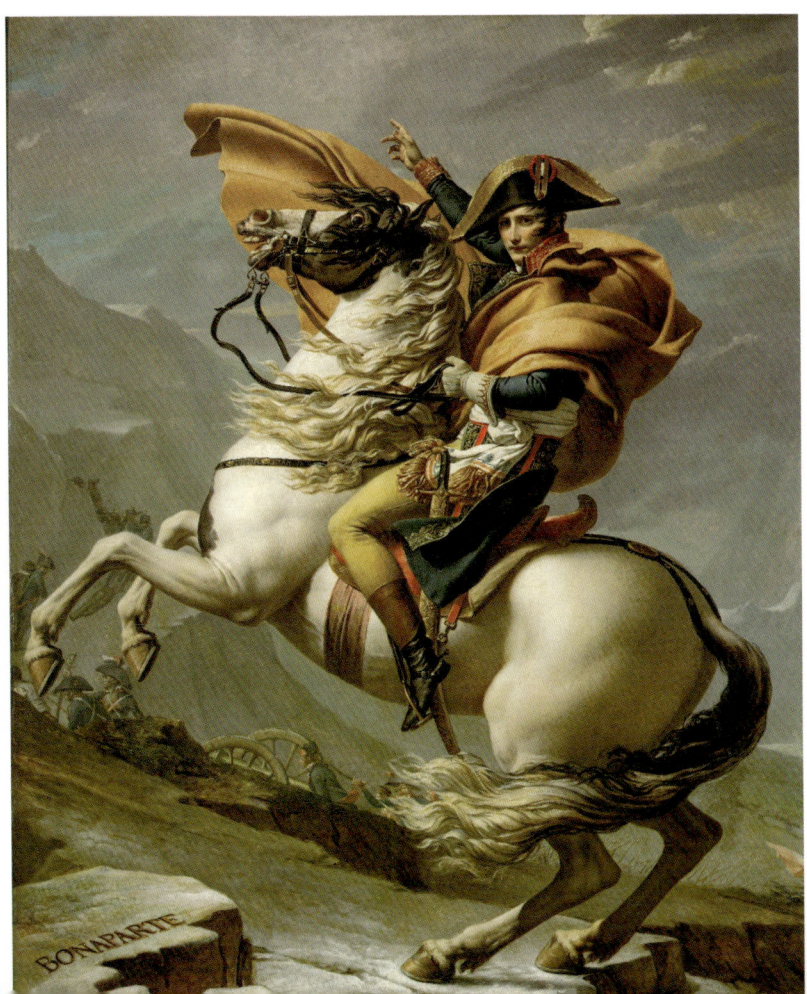

epilepsy, for example. Artist Vincent van Gogh and Lewis Carroll, the author of *Alice's Adventures in Wonderland,* also lived with the disorder.

Just as epileptics can become famous politicians and artists, most can do all the things that make up more ordinary lives. Epileptics, for example, can attend school and college, participate in sports, and have a wide range of employment opportunities open to them. One area of life where epileptics may have less freedom than others, however, is in driving automobiles.

Driving Can Be Dangerous

Most countries have laws regarding epilepsy and driving. In the United States, six states have laws that require doctors to inform state health officials when their patients suffer from epileptic seizures. These health officials feel that drivers with epilepsy put themselves, their passengers, and other drivers and pedestrians at risk if they drive when their seizures are not under control. An epileptic seizure might cause a driver to lose consciousness, for example, and cause an accident. For this reason, states like California ask people with active epileptic seizures to give up their driver's licenses until they can prove they have not had a seizure for a year.

Because so many people rely on their cars for a sense of freedom and for getting to work each day, some drivers with epilepsy do not report their

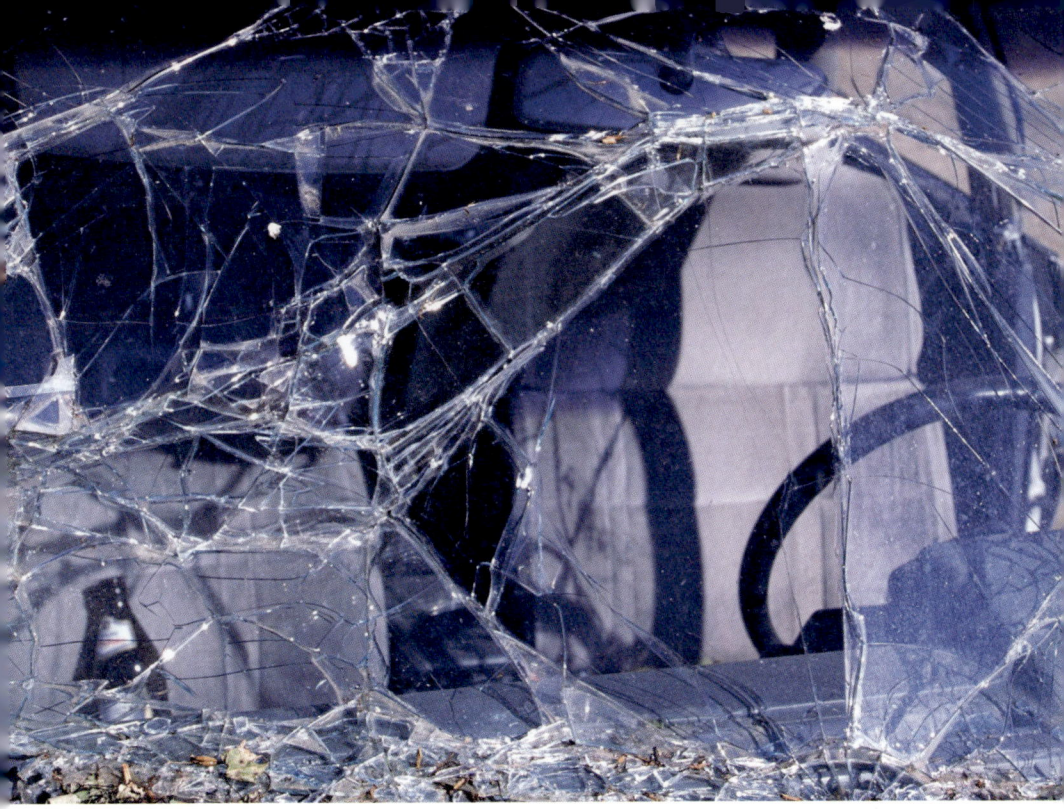

An epileptic driver who loses consciousness during a seizure can cause a horrible accident.

seizures to their doctors because they fear their licenses will be taken away. *Los Angeles Times* staff writer Jane E. Allen reports that a 1993 Stanford University survey found that out of 400 adults with epilepsy, 207 people admitted not telling their doctors about seizures in the past. Of these patients, 86 percent said they did not want to lose their driver's licenses.

Overall, this study concluded that four out of five epileptics would stop driving if their seizures were not under control. But health officials are still concerned about those who are withholding information from their doctors. "We can't properly

Living with Epilepsy

treat people if we don't know if or when they're having seizures,"⁵ said Kamala Rodrigues, one of the neurologists who conducted the research.

Children with Epilepsy Have Special Concerns

Children with epilepsy can have special concerns as well. These children are more likely than other children to have learning disabilities and behavioral and emotional problems, for example. In school, classmates may not understand that epilepsy is not a disease they can catch. They might also become afraid when their peers with epilepsy have seizures at school.

Children with epilepsy are more likely than other children to develop behavioral and emotional problems.

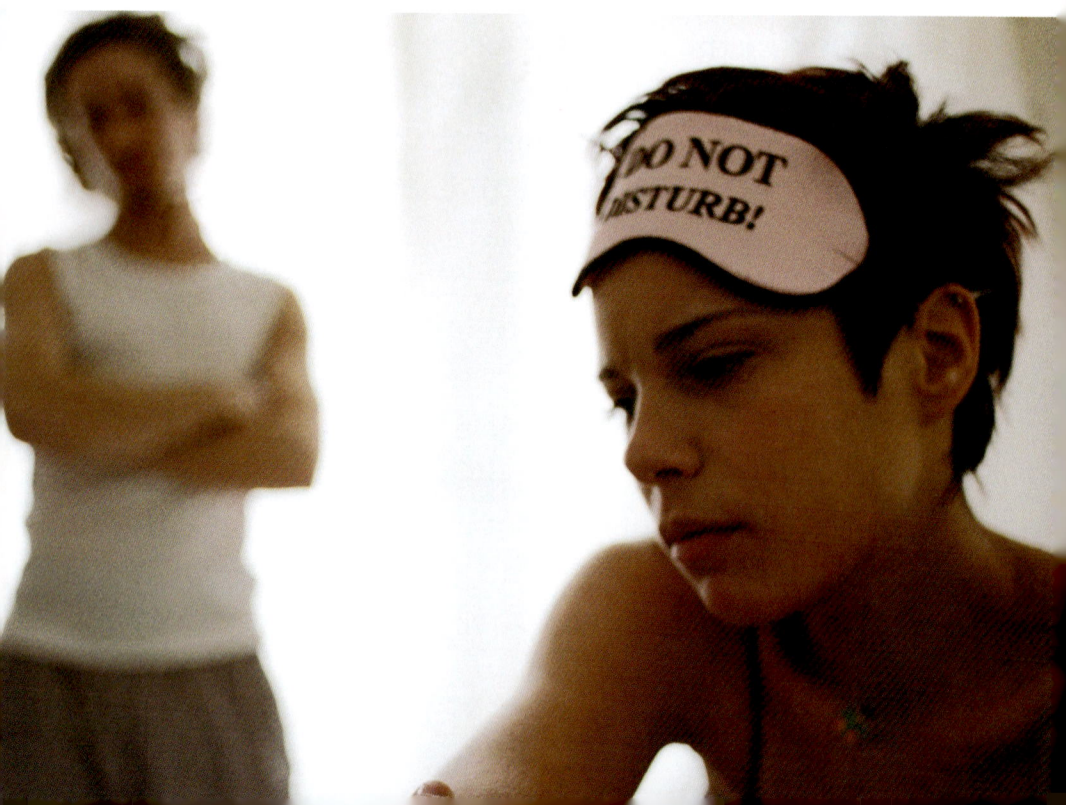

One school nurse says, "I think in general the public is more aware of, and sympathetic to, seizure disorders than twenty years ago. However, we need to work at dispelling fear: fear of having to deal with a seizure, and fear of the person who has seizures."[6] Because of this fear, children with epilepsy are often teased by their peers, bullied, or excluded from group activities outside of class.

Behavior Limits and Peer Perceptions

Alysa Mendes is an eighteen-year-old in Tennessee who has had epileptic seizures at school. Although she often does not remember her seizures, she knows she has had one, she says, when "I wake up, and either everybody in the school is standing around me, or I'm in an ambulance."[7] Unlike many other teens, Alysa has not been teased at school because of her epilepsy, but she does feel her condition limits the kinds of things she is allowed to do. For example, she is not allowed to attend sleepovers unless she is with a friend who knows what to do during a seizure.

Alysa's parents and closest friends have become protective of her because of her epilepsy. "If I'm sick at all, like if I have a cold, people freak out," she says. "It's frustrating because I don't want to be different from everybody, but on the other hand, it's nice to know they care."[8] One of Alysa's friends, Katherine, cares so much about her that she has worked with Alysa to help correct their peers' misunderstandings about epilepsy.

Students Are Learning About Epilepsy

Alysa and Katherine have distributed brochures and educational materials about epilepsy at their school and in their community. They have also raised money for the Epilepsy Foundation of East Tennessee in Alysa's name by sponsoring movie nights and car washes. Alysa's and Katherine's efforts have helped give their peers a better understanding about epilepsy, but nationwide, most kids know very little about the disorder. Kristi L. Nelson, health writer for the *Knoxville News-Sentinel* reported in 2002 that according to the Epilepsy Foundation, of 19,441 American teens surveyed, "nearly half had not heard of epilepsy or thought it may be contagious (it's not). Nearly one in five said epilepsy is a mental illness; 52 percent said people die from seizures."[9]

Like Alysa and Katherine, however, the foundation has taken steps to increase kids' awareness about epilepsy through its new campaign, "Entitled to Respect." With the support of the pop group *NSYNC, which allows the foundation to use pictures of band members, the Epilepsy Foundation has distributed informational brochures and posters in schools, libraries, shopping malls, and coffee shops. These materials teach kids

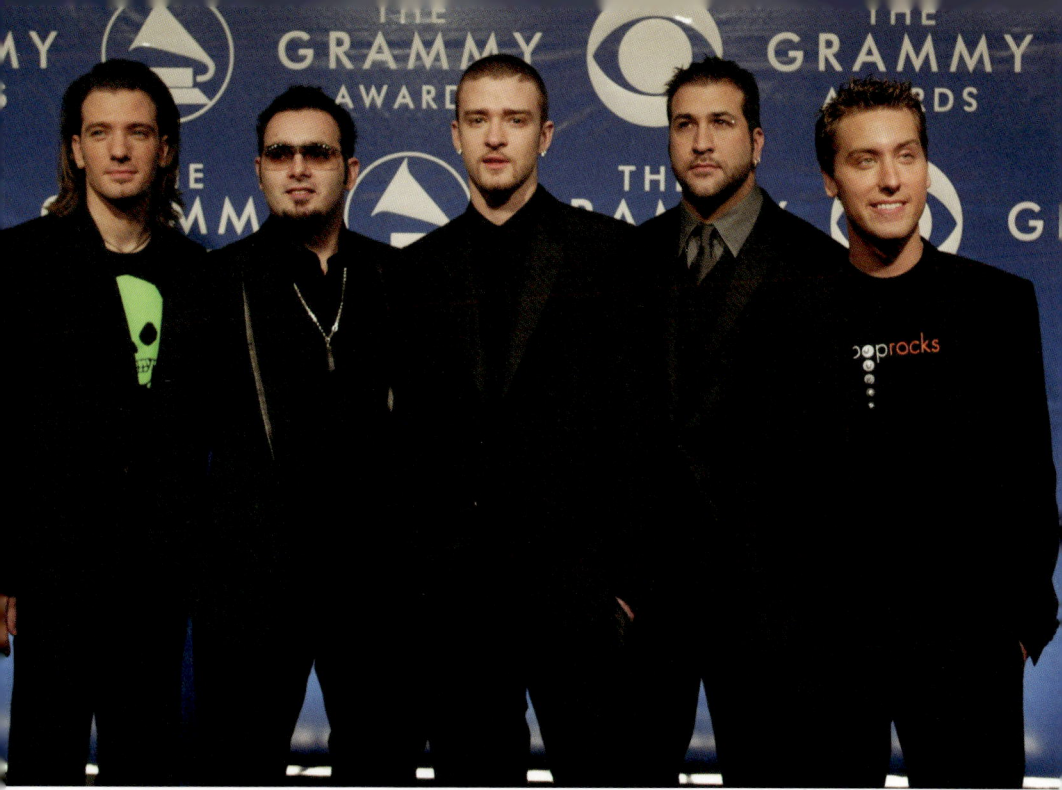

The pop group *NSYNC is helping the Epilepsy Foundation to teach kids about epilepsy.

about epilepsy and encourage them to be respectful of their peers with epilepsy.

Lynn Goad, the education coordinator for the Epilepsy Foundation of East Tennessee, feels this campaign and educational programs about epilepsy are steps in the right direction. "The lack of information out there is amazing," she says. "A surprising number of kids report that they've seen a seizure, but almost none can tell us anything about epilepsy."[10] Because of this lack of understanding, Goad's group has given over 130 educational presentations on epilepsy to nearly five thousand students in East Tennessee middle and high schools.

Living with Epilepsy

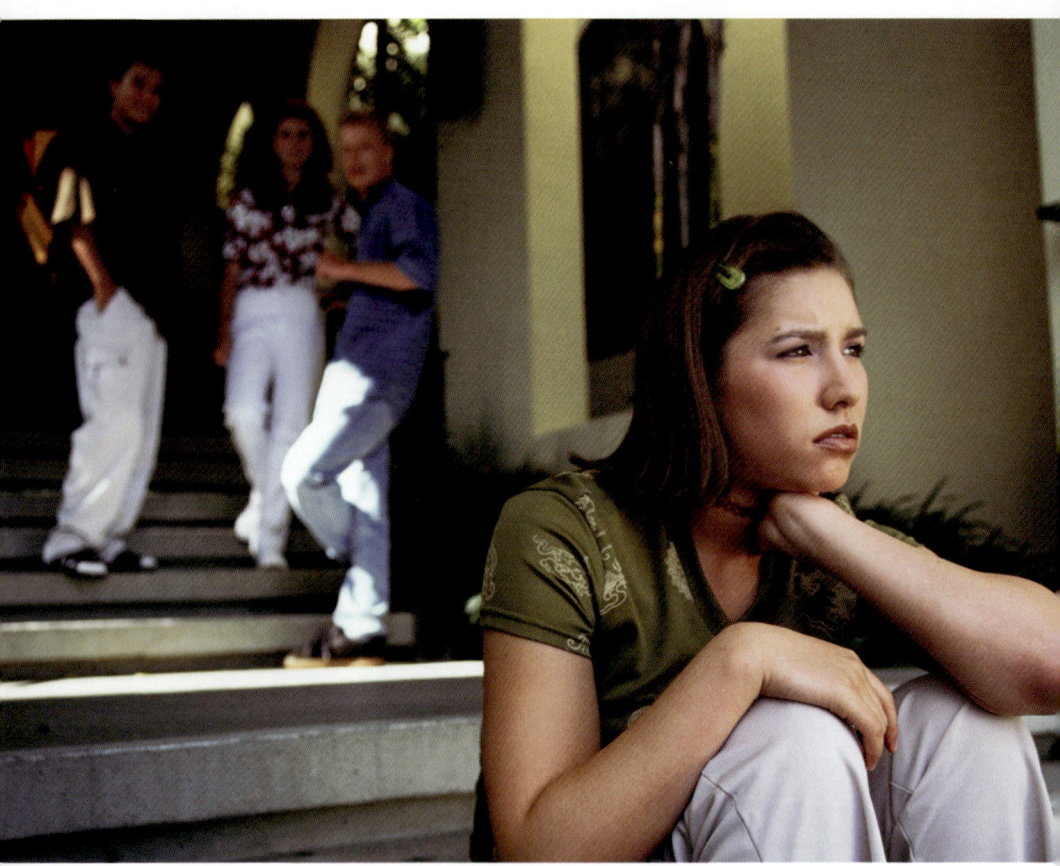

Being excluded from a group because of epilepsy is hurtful.

Kids Take Epilepsy Concerns to Congress

Schoolchildren are not only learning about epilepsy; some are teaching adults about the disorder. Frustrated by most people's lack of understanding about epilepsy and the medical and social consequences of having the disorder, thirty-eight children with epilepsy from twenty-five states went to Capitol Hill in April 2003 to ask Congress and the Senate for support. As part of the Epilepsy Foundation's "Kids Speak Up" program, these kids are asking for funding for more health education about epilepsy in their schools. They also want members of Congress to renew their pledge for continuing medical research on epilepsy.

Linda Warner is a parent whose child has epilepsy. She is also the chair of the Epilepsy Foundation. She often reminds people that "Children with epilepsy suffer greatly when school communities do not understand them. Misconceptions and isolation can be just as painful emotionally as the seizures themselves."[11] She thinks the "Kids Speak Up" program offers a good opportunity for the public to learn more about this condition. Fortunately for these children and others with epilepsy, it can be treated.

Chapter Four

Treating Epilepsy

While more education may help cure some people's fear of epilepsy, there are, fortunately, a number of ways to treat the disease. In fact, up to 80 percent of people with the condition can control their epilepsy with medication.

Drug Therapy Often Works

The main goal of doctors treating epilepsy is to stop seizures or to make the symptoms less frequent and less severe. The most common way to do this is through the use of long-term **anticonvulsant drug** therapy. Anticonvulsant drugs act on the brain to either prevent epileptics from having seizures or to help make seizures less severe. Patients who begin treatment with these drugs are often required to take them for the rest of their lives to control their epilepsy.

People who are taking anticonvulsant drugs need to be monitored frequently by their doctors to test for the amounts of the drugs that remain in their bloodstream. A simple blood test shows whether a patient's blood has changed or if his or her liver has been negatively affected by the drugs. Some signs that too much of the drug has entered the bloodstream include uncontrolled eye movements, sluggishness, dizziness, hyperactivity, vomiting, or trouble sleeping.

Blood tests allow doctors to monitor the condition of their epileptic patients who take anticonvulsant drugs.

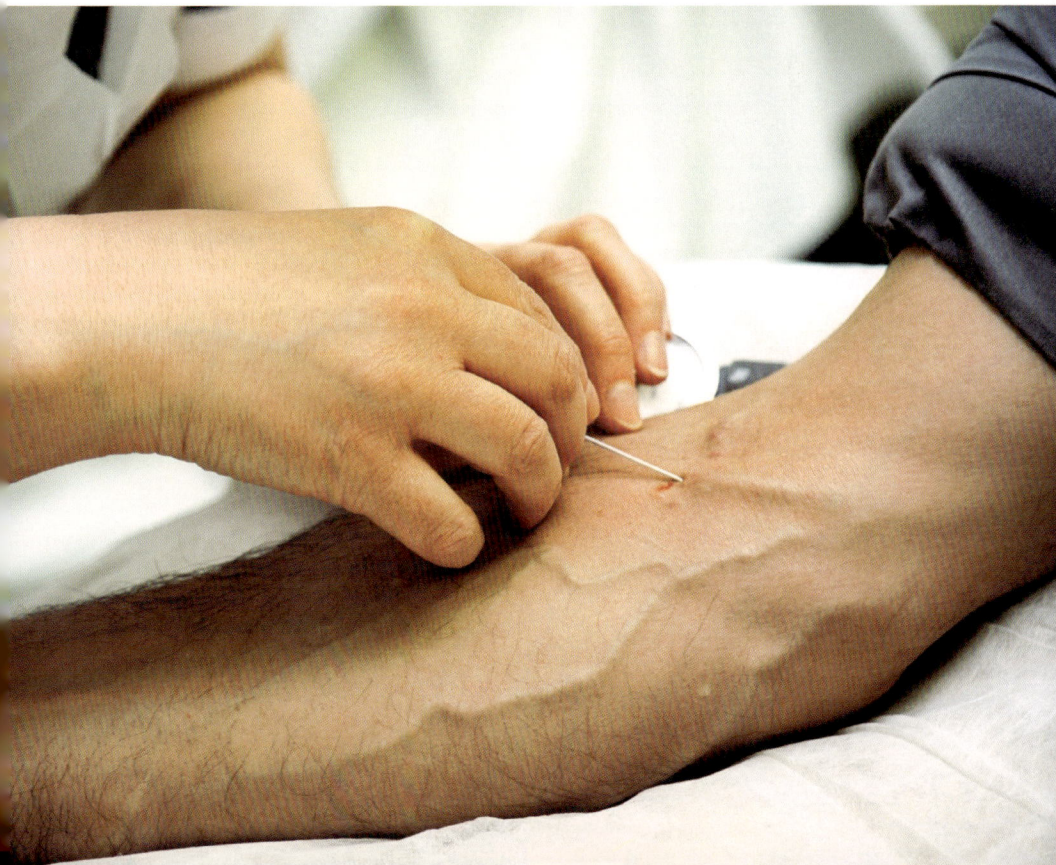

Negative side effects are common when taking medication of any kind, and the same holds true for anticonvulsant drugs. Many of these drugs are addictive, for example, and they can cause nausea, drowsiness, or dizziness, and make people feel less alert. Anticonvulsants may also increase a patient's sensitivity to sunlight, so that even brief sun exposure can result in a sunburn. Fortunately, most of these side effects are short-term. Many patients only experience them while their doctors are working to find out how much of the anticonvulsant medicine they need.

The Natural Approach to Treating Epilepsy

Some patients find that natural approaches to treatment help improve their conditions. The most common natural therapies for epilepsy are those that help relieve stress and encourage relaxation. Yoga, hypnosis, meditation, and massage, for example, are all stress-relieving natural therapies.

In addition to relaxing, many epilepsy patients also change their eating habits. A diet rich in whole foods, such as fresh fruits and vegetables, and light in processed foods, such as frozen or fast foods, is often beneficial to the health of epilepsy patients. Some patients, especially those whose epilepsy has not responded to drugs, choose to follow an even more extreme diet plan. Under the care of their physicians, they are put on a **ketogenic diet.**

Unlike a diet for weight loss that is low in fat, a ketogenic diet is high in the kinds of fats found in meats, cheeses, butter, and cream. But it is low in carbohydrates found in bread, cereal, and grains. This diet changes the body's chemistry and the way it converts food into energy by increasing the blood's supply of the chemicals called ketones. This increased supply of ketones suppresses seizures in many patients, but it does not work for everyone. The diet is most successful for children under age ten, and doctors need to watch for negative side effects such as stunted growth, low blood sugar, and excess fat in the blood.

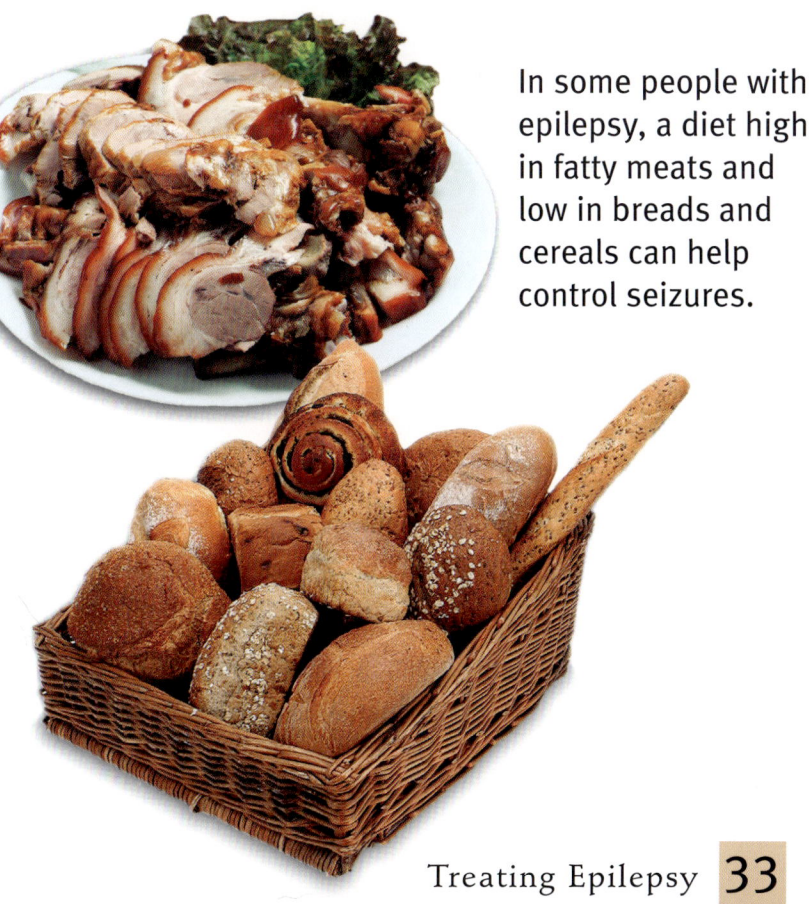

In some people with epilepsy, a diet high in fatty meats and low in breads and cereals can help control seizures.

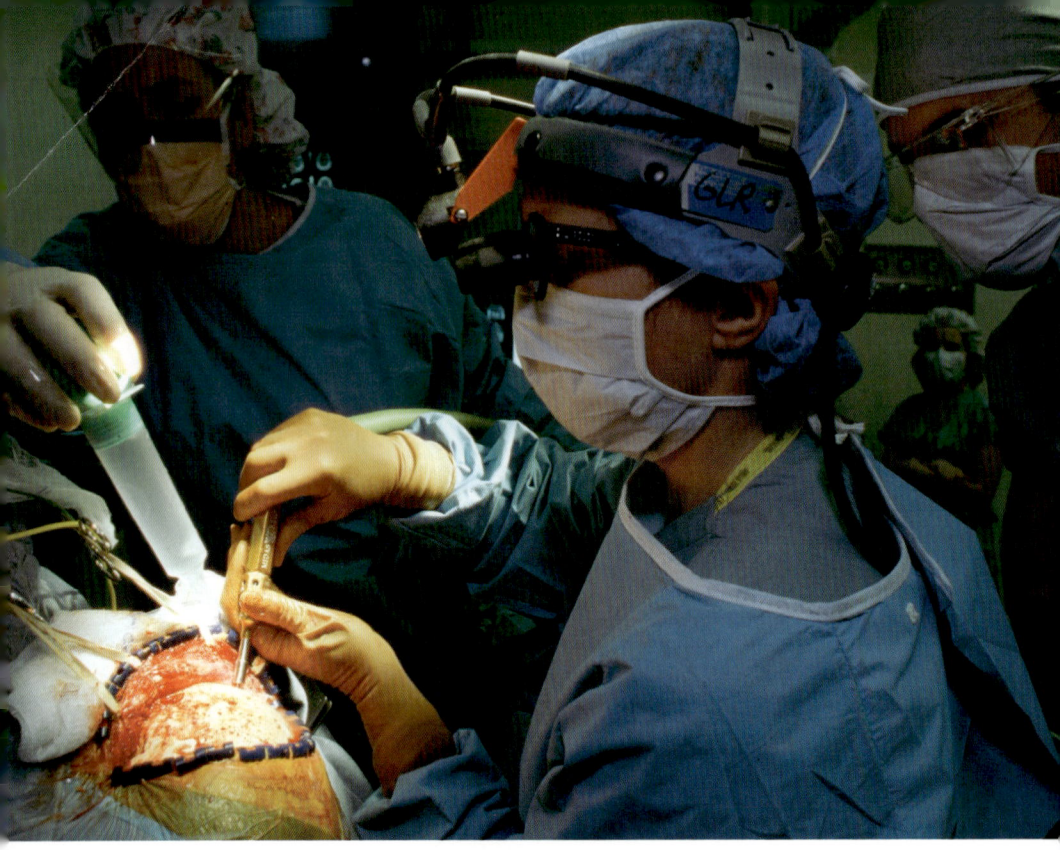

A team of surgeons performs brain surgery to cure the seizures of an epileptic.

Surgery Can Cure Seizures

Epilepsy patients who find no relief for their seizures through drug treatment or the ketogenic diet may turn to surgery. Lesionectomy and temporal lobectomy are two examples of brain surgeries performed to cure epileptic seizures. Epilepsy patients whose seizures are caused by small lesions in the brain can have them removed in surgery. This process, called lesionectomy, does not endanger the patient or change his or her personality or ability to function normally.

Another effective brain surgery to control epileptic seizures is the temporal lobectomy. In this procedure, doctors remove a small portion of the **temporal lobe** responsible for partial seizures, the kind that only occur in one part of the brain. Of the patients who choose this surgery, 75 to 85 percent have no further seizures. Of the remaining patients, 90 percent have fewer seizures than before the surgery.

Epilepsy patients often turn to surgery only as a last resort, but a 2001 clinical study suggests that surgery should be performed more frequently. In fact, the study found that at least 100,000 of the 2 million Americans with epilepsy might benefit from surgery. However, only 1,500 epileptics seek surgical treatment each year.

"What makes this study significant is that, for the first time, we have a strong prospective study that clearly shows the value of epilepsy surgery," said Dr. Gregory L. Barkley of the Henry Ford Comprehensive Epilepsy Program in Detroit. "The bottom line is that, if you've tried several drug combinations for a year to a year and a half, then you should think about surgery so that the patients can get on with their lives."[12]

Dale's Brain Surgery

Dale is a thirty-year-old man who has had epilepsy since he was ten years old. In July 2002 he opted to have surgery to help control his seizures. He discusses his experience with his surgery on his Web site.

Like many epilepsy patients who choose surgery, Dale noticed some side effects soon after the treatment. In his case, he felt the nerves in his face were not functioning normally. "Touch my right side of my lip and I feel all across my cheek," he writes. "Touch my cheek and I feel it on my lips (as well as on my cheek). Touch my nose and I feel it on my eyebrow. Scratch my forehead and I feel it up on my head."[13]

In addition to experiencing these side effects, Dale discovered that despite the surgery, his seizures did not stop completely. He says, however, that compared to the many seizures he was having an hour, now whole days will pass without his having one. Because of this, he says that for him the surgery was worth it.

What to Do if Someone Has a Seizure

No matter what therapy people with epilepsy choose, they will still experience seizures from time to time. Just as treatment options are important for these patients, it is also important for them to have people around them who know what to do when a seizure does hit. Fortunately, there are a number of things people can do to help make their friends' and family members' seizures less traumatic.

People who experience petit mal seizures rarely need help from others, as these episodes often go unnoticed. On the other hand, people who have grand mal seizures often need assistance. Convulsions occur in grand mal seizures, and people who experience them often lose consciousness. For this reason, people suffering from a grand mal seizure may need help to avoid hitting their arms, legs, and especially heads on the floor, furniture, or other obstructions.

After helping someone suffering a grand mal seizure to the floor, no one should attempt to restrain the person. The seizure cannot be stopped

First Aid for a Grand Mal Seizure

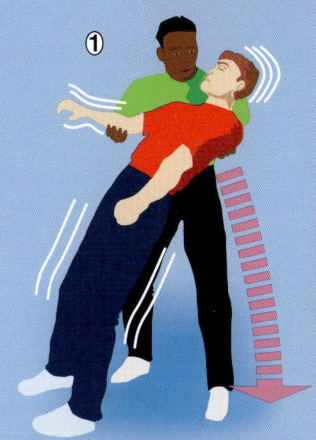

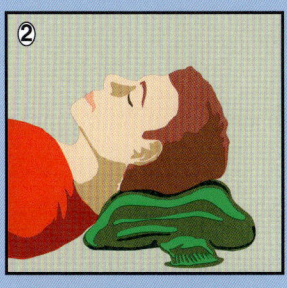

① Help the person to the floor. **Do not hold him or her down.**

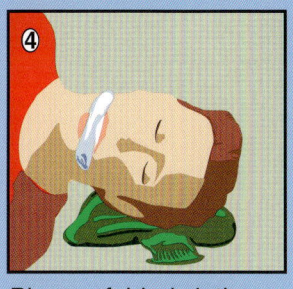

② Place something soft under the head.

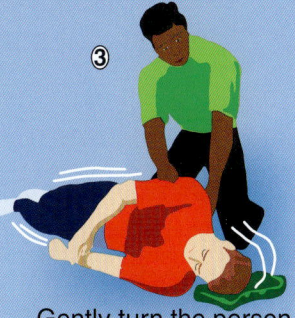

③ Gently turn the person on his or her side.

④ Place a folded cloth in the person's mouth.

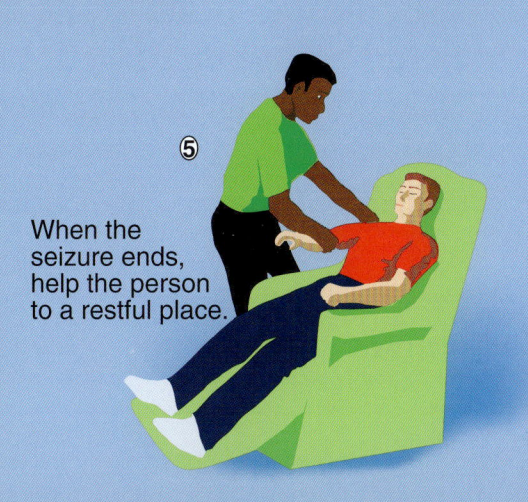

⑤ When the seizure ends, help the person to a restful place.

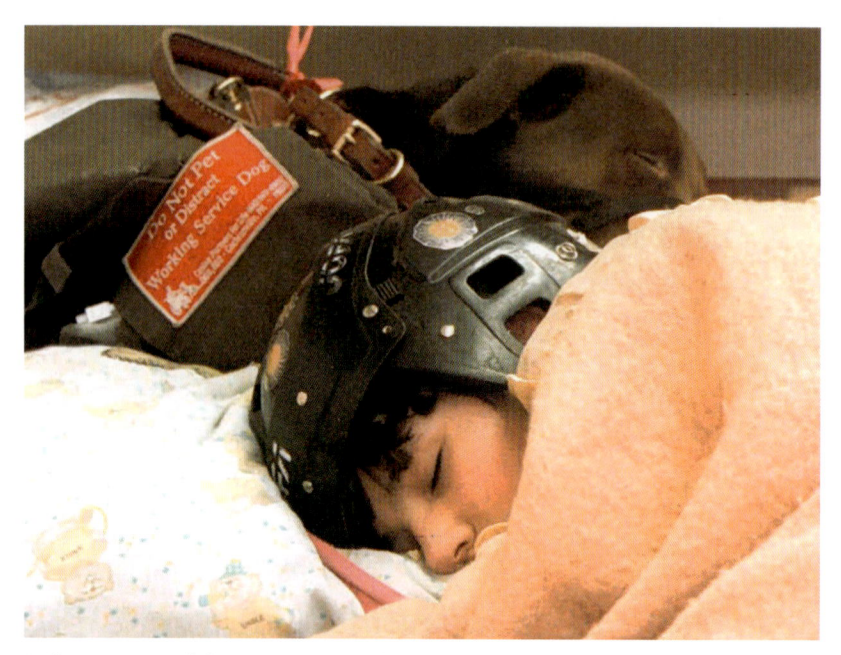

Whenever this young epileptic is about to have a seizure, a specially trained dog alerts her to wear a helmet that protects her head.

by holding the person down, and trying to do so may cause injury. The person can be made more comfortable, however, by placing a pillow, towel, or other soft object under his or her head. It is also helpful to move the person onto one side. This helps the tongue fall to one side in the mouth and creates an open passage for air into the person's body. Those helping can also place a folded soft cloth into the person's mouth to prevent the tongue from being bitten during the seizure. Hard objects, however, should never be placed in the person's mouth as they can cause injury or obstruct breathing.

After experiencing grand mal seizures, people with epilepsy are likely to be disoriented and confused. They should be gently told that they have suffered a seizure and reminded where they are, so they do not become frightened. Rarely will people suffering from grand mal seizures need to seek immediate medical attention. Thus ambulances should only be called if they do not start breathing after a seizure, if they have repeated seizures, or if they become injured as a result of convulsions.

Finally, people who have suffered grand mal seizures should be helped to a place where they can rest until the effects of the seizures have worn off. All of these steps will help people with grand mal seizures make it safely through their epileptic episodes. Those with epilepsy also appreciate when others around them do not look upon their seizures with fear and embarrassment but with compassion and understanding.

Notes

Chapter 1: What Is Epilepsy?
1. Quoted in Epilepsy Action, "Ben's Story," www.epilepsy.org.uk/kids/index.html.
2. Quoted in Robert J. Michael, *The Educator's Guide to Students with Epilepsy.* Springfield, IL: Charles C. Thomas, 1995, p. 19.

Chapter 2: What Causes Epilepsy?
3. Catlina, "Personal Stories: Out of the Blue," Epilepsy Foundation, September 7, 2003. www.epilepsyfoundation.org/e2r/stories.cfm.
4. Catlina, "Personal Stories: Out of the Blue."

Chapter 3: Living with Epilepsy
5. Quoted in Jane E. Allen, "Medicine: Drivers Not Telling Doctors of Seizures; Some Report Concealing Episodes Because They Don't Want to Lose Their Licenses, a Survey Finds," *Los Angeles Times,* April 7, 2003, p. F3.
6. Quoted in Michael, *The Educator's Guide to Students with Epilepsy,* p. 138.

7. Quoted in Kristi L. Nelson, "Active but Aware; with Friends' Help, Epileptic Teenagers Lead Normal Lives," *Knoxville News-Sentinel*, November 12, 2001, p. E1.
8. Quoted in Nelson, "Active but Aware," p. E1.
9. Nelson, "Active but Aware," p. E1.
10. Quoted in Nelson, "Active but Aware," p. E1.
11. Quoted in PR Newswire Association, "Children from 25 States Seek Congressional Support in Dealing with Epilepsy," April 7, 2003.

Chapter 4: Treating Epilepsy

12. Quoted in Thomas H. Maugh II, "Surgery Viable for Epilepsy," *Los Angeles Times,* August 2, 2001, p. A9.
13. "Surgery Is Fun: Dale's Surgery," www.hugger.net/brainsurgery.

Glossary

anticonvulsant drug: A drug developed to control the occurrence of epileptic seizures.

convulsion: A repeated tightening of muscles and jerking of limbs.

epilepsy: A chronic disorder of the brain resulting in the tendency to have recurrent seizures.

generalized seizure: One of two types of epileptic seizures, generalized seizures spread throughout the entire brain rather than remaining focused in one area.

grand mal seizure: Also known as generalized tonic-clonic seizure; a person having this kind of seizure becomes unconscious and falls, and the body stiffens and jerks with convulsions.

ketogenic diet: A high-fat, low carbohydrate diet that changes the process by which the body converts food to energy; it controls generalized seizures in children.

neuron: A cell of the brain and nervous system specialized to transmit information in the form of tiny electrical impulses.

partial seizure: A seizure that remains localized in the area of the brain from which it originated.

petit mal seizure: A seizure in which a person stares blankly and loses touch with his or her surroundings for a few moments.

seizure: A sudden discharge of excess electricity within the brain that causes a momentary shift in behavior.

stroke: The sudden blockage of blood circulation to the brain or part of the brain; can result in epilepsy.

temporal lobe: The area of the brain that controls memory; the most common site of partial seizures.

For Further Exploration

Books

Nonfiction

Mark Edward Dudley, *Epilepsy*. Springfield, NJ: Enslow, 2001. This book discusses the causes, diagnosis, and treatment of epilepsy, the types of seizures, and the challenges of living with the disease.

Patricia Emmanuel, *Everything You Need to Know About Epilepsy*. New York: Rosen, 2000. The goal of this book is to dispel myths and misunderstandings about epilepsy, in addition to offering young readers advice on how to live with this condition.

Sally Fletcher, *The Challenge of Epilepsy*. Santa Rosa, CA: Aura, 1985. An easy-to-read guide meant to instruct, encourage, and inspire epileptics.

Melanie Apel Gordon, *Let's Talk Epilepsy*. New York: Rosen, 2003. This author explains the nature, causes, symptoms, and treatment of epilepsy.

Shirley Wimbish Gray, *Living with Epilepsy*. Portsmouth, NH: Child's World, 2002. This text provides insight into the condition of epilepsy, while offering a detailed account of what it is like to live with this disorder.

Elaine Landau, *Epilepsy*. New York: Twenty-First Century Books, 1994. This book offers a very basic introduction to epilepsy and is written for young readers.

Andrew N. Wilner, *Epilepsy: 199 Answers: A Doctor Responds to His Patients' Questions*. Boston: Demos Medical, 1996. An encyclopedic reference of the disorder, and a good resource for people of all ages with and without epilepsy.

Fiction

Rachel Anderson, *Black Water*. Baltimore: PaperStar Books, 1996. Written for young readers, this book approaches epilepsy from a historical angle. It provides details in the life of a young epileptic boy in nineteenth-century England.

Laurie Lears, *Becky the Brave: A Story About Epilepsy*. Morton Grove, IL: Albert Whitman, 2002. Sarah's big sister Becky is afraid to return to school after having an epileptic seizure. Sarah helps make it easier for Becky by explaining epilepsy to the other students before her return.

Web Sites

EpiCentre (http://ourworld.compuserve.com). This well-designed site covers all the introductory basics of epilepsy, from definitions to causes to treatment.

Epilepsy.com (www.epilepsy.com). The goal of this site is to empower epilepsy patients and their families. It provides in-depth information about epilepsy in a format accessible to nonprofessionals.

Epilepsy Foundation (www.efa.org). Sponsored by the largest epilepsy support group in America, this site provides personal perspectives on epilepsy, and information on modern research and advances in treatment. The site also includes links to other epilepsy-related sites.

KidsHealth (http://kidshealth.org/kid/health-problems/epilepsy.html). This site offers basic information about epilepsy in an easy-to-follow format. It highlights people living with epilepsy and stresses that they are able to live happy, productive lives.

Index

alcohol, 18–19
Allen, Jane E., 23
anticonvulsant drugs, 30–32

Barkley, Gregory L., 35
behavior, 15–17, 24
Ben, 6
body chemistry, 33
brain
  control of daily functions by, 4–5
  injuries to, 13, 14
  surgeries, 24–26

Caesar, Julius, 21–22
California, 22
Carroll, Lewis, 22
Catlina, 15–17
cerebral cortex, 4
childbirth trauma, 13
childhood diseases, 13
children
  ketogenic diet and, 33
  special concerns of, 24–27
consciousness, loss of, 10, 12, 37
convulsions, 5, 37

Dale, 35–36
diet, 16, 17, 32–33
driving, 22–24
drugs, 19, 30–32

eating habits, 16, 17, 32–33
"Entitled to Respect," 26
Epilepsy Foundation, 26, 29

flickering lights, 15

generalized seizures, 8, 9
Goad, Lynn, 27
grand mal seizures, 9–10, 12, 37–39

health education, 26–27, 29

hypnosis, 32

incidence, 7, 15

Katherine, 25–26
ketogenic diet, 32–33
"Kids Speak Up," 29

learning disabilities, 24
lesionectomy, 34

massage, 32
medications, 19, 30–32
meditation, 32
Mendes, Alysa, 25–26
Michael, Robert J., 10

Napoléon, 21–22
Nelson, Kristi L., 26
neurons, 4–5
*NSYNC, 26

partial seizures, 8–9
Peter the Great, 21–22
petit mal seizures, 10, 12, 36
photosensitivity, 15
poisons, 13–14
precautions, 21

relaxation, 32
Rodrigues, Kamala, 23–24

seizures
  alcohol and drug triggers of, 18–19
  behavioral triggers of, 15–17
  brain trauma and, 13, 14
  disease triggers of, 13
  helping during, 36–39
  neurons and, 4–5
  symptoms during, 5, 7
  types of, 8–10, 12, 36
sleep, lack of, 15
stress, 15
strokes, 14–15
surgeries, 24–26
Susan, 10

temporal lobectomy, 35
treatment
  drug therapy, 30–32
  natural approaches, 32–33
  surgeries, 24–26

U. S. Congress, 28–29

van Gogh, Vincent, 22

Warner, Linda, 29
warning signals, 16, 20

yoga, 32